ESSENTIAL OILS FOR ALLERGIES

Out of the Box Approach to eliminate
your allergies with essential Oils

Tonny M Ford, RN, BSN, PHN

© 2015

Essential Oils

FOR ALLERGIES

AN OUT OF THE BOX APPROACH TO ELIMINATE YOUR ALLERGIES WITH ESSENTIAL OILS

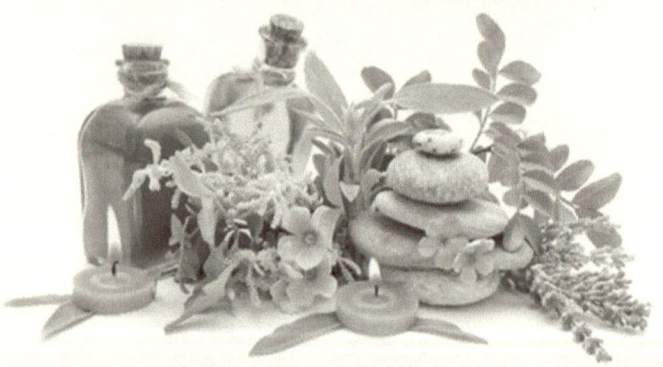

TONNY M FORD, RN, BSN, PHN

essentialoilRN.net

Disclaimer

This book is not intended as a substitute for the medical advice of physicians. The reader should regularly consult a physician in matters relating to his/her health and particularly with respect to any symptoms that may require diagnosis or medical attention.

The information provided in this book is designed to provide helpful information on the subjects discussed. This book is not meant to be used, nor should it be used, to diagnose or treat any medical condition. For diagnosis or treatment of any medical problem, consult your own physician. The publisher and author are not responsible for any specific health or medical needs that may require medical supervision and are not liable for any damages or negative consequences from any treatment, action, application or preparation, to any person reading or following the information in this book. References are provided for informational purposes only and do not constitute endorsement of any websites or other sources. Readers should be aware that the websites listed in this book may change.

We highly recommend that you consult a doctor and other trained clinicians before using essentials oils or anything that can affect your health. Your doctor is the only one who know the true story of your health and can give your better professional help.

TABLE OF CONTENTS

Introduction

I want to thank you and congratulate you for owning the book, *"Essential Oils for Allergies: An Out of the Box Approach to eliminate your allergies with essential Oils"*.
This book was designed to give you all the information you need to treat common allergies naturally with essential oils.

Essential oils are an organic, all-natural and safer alternative to many potentially dangerous products and drugs that we come in contact with on a daily basis. The truth is, many common items that we inhale, ingest and put onto our bodies can cause more harm than good. Thankfully, many of these products can be replaced with essential oils, as we will discuss in this book.

If you follow the instructions in this book and use the essential oils as described, you will notice an improvement in your allergy systems as well as a positive effect on your overall health and well-being. Keep in mind, however, that you shouldn't use essential oils all willy-nilly. You should first do your research since some essential oils shouldn't be used by children, if you suffer from certain medical conditions or are pregnant or nursing. If, however, you do your due diligence, you will reap the many benefits provided by essential oils.

Thanks again for purchasing this book, I hope you enjoy it!

Chapter 1 – The Basic of Essential Oils

While the words 'essential oils' are common in today's day in age, not everyone knows exactly what essential oils are. Essential oils are volatile liquids that are derived from plants. Essential oils can come from many different parts of plants, including the flowers, seeds, leaves, fruit, roots, barks and stems.

Essential oils contain a wide array of chemical constituents, including alcohols, ketones, terpenes, esters, phenols and aldehydes. And all these chemical constituents can be effected by various facts, such as where the plant came from, the fertilizer used in the growing process, soil condition, altitude, climate, geographical region, method used to harvest and what process of distillation was used.

For thousands of years, essential oils have been used for their medicinal properties. In the

Christian Bible alone, there are about 188 references to the use of essential oils. In fact, you can find references to essential oils in many ancient texts.

Essential Oil Benefits

Essential oils are beneficial because they contain medicinal and healing properties. And since they are derived from plants, they are considered natural, organic and a safer alternative to chemical treatment and cures. Essential oils have immune enhancing abilities and support various body systems, including the immune, respiratory, circulatory, digestive, endocrine and nervous system. Essential oils are also high in antioxidants and have oxygenating and antiseptic properties. Furthermore, essential oils can lift spirits, relax your body, calm your mind and give you energy. As if that wasn't enough positive aspects, essential oils are extremely aromatic with pleasant scents and can fill your home and life with a natural, non-chemical aroma.

Essential Oil Quality Is Vital

In order to have the most beneficial essential oil, you will need 100-percent pure, unadulterated oil. Pure essential oil occurs when the delicate compounds of the essential oil is preserved as much as possible. Excessive pressure and high temperatures will destroy these delicate compounds, as will chemically reactive metals, like aluminum and copper.

You can use essential oils alone or combine them with other essential oils. No matter what you use them for, you must make sure to only use high quality oils. There are some companies, unfortunately, that will manufacture poor quality oils that used a high heat distillation or chemical extraction. What this does is cause the medicinal properties and healthy benefits of the essential oil to become compromised. In essence, low quality oils are useless and have little to no medicinal benefits.

It's surprising to many that the FDA (Food and Drug Administration) only requires 10-percent of the essential oil to be "pure essential oil". That is why you should do your research and purchase only 100-percent pure food or therapeutic grade essential oil.

Essential Oil Uses

Besides health benefits, essential oils can be used to create your very own healthy body and bath products, organic pet care items and safe household cleaners. You can even use essential oils for culinary purposes or to make non-chemical fragrances for your home or your body.

Considerations

If you are not sure how an essential oil can benefit you, your health and your family, simply research the plant that the oil is derived from and what health benefits it has. Each essential oil provides various benefits that can improve many different aspects of your life.

This information is readily available in various books and even for free online.

With the basic information found in this book, anyone can safely jump start their new journey into the wonderful world of essential oils.

Chapter 2 – Allergies: What You Need to Know

Thirty to 40-percent of the entire population suffers from some type of allergy or allergy-related disease, according to the World Health Organization (WHO). Allergies are one of the most common ailments that people of all ages can deal with.

An allergic reaction occurs when the immune system reacts to foreign substances entering the body. I know this definition sounds a bit vague, but the truth is that a person can be allergic to just about anything. This is because everything outside your body is a foreign substance. From the food you eat, the drinks you ingest and the air particles you breathe, these can trigger an allergy attack in those who are allergic to that certain substance. Now, it is not the actual substance that is causing the problem. It is the way your body identifies the substance as harmful, thus making it an allergen.

Respiratory Reaction

When the substance you are allergic to enters the respiratory system, it causes cold-like symptoms. This is typically called hay fever and generally occurs in the spring and fall when plants and vegetation are pollinating and decaying. Hay fever is one of the most common types of allergic reactions. This is because it is almost impossible to avoid.

Some of the most common symptoms associated with respiratory allergies are:

- Stuffy or runny nose
- Sneezing
- Irritated eyes (red, itchy, swollen watery)
- Wheezing

Food Reactions

Food is another common cause of allergies. However, food allergies are typically more severe and serious in nature than respiratory allergies. Unfortunately, many mild food allergies go undiagnosed because people don't associate the reaction with their food. Celiac disease and lactose intolerance are two types of food allergies that should be diagnosed as early as possible because of the extreme discomfort the cause the sufferer.

Some of the most common symptoms associated with food allergies are:

- Tingling in the mouth
- Swollen tongue, lips and/or face
- Nausea

If any of these symptoms regularly occur after consuming a certain type of food, you should consult with your doctor as soon as possible to find out if you are having an allergic reaction.

Skin Reactions

Just about anything can cause a skin reaction. Exposure to grass, bee sting, reaction to a vaccination, a mosquito bite, or something you consumed; these are just a few things that can lead to a skin reaction. Your skin acts like a barometer that lets you know if you have touched or ingested something that you shouldn't have.

Some of the most common symptoms associated with skin allergies are:

- Itchy skin
- Rash Hives
- Peeling or flaking skin
- Swelling around the area of skin exposed

If you notice a bump, flaking or rash, try to determine what caused the reaction. It could actually be a cause of more serious skin allergy.

Potentially Fatal Reactions

Some people suffer from an allergy that could cause a fatal reaction, which is called anaphylaxis. Unfortunately, it is hard to know beforehand if someone's immune system will have such an extreme reaction that it puts their life in danger. Because of this, certain social events and schools are affected. For example, a nut allergy is a common allergen that can be potentially fatal, causing the throat to close up, which leads to suffocation. The person having the extreme reaction will often go into shock and lose consciousness.

Some of the most common symptoms associated with anaphylactic shock are:

- Drastic drop in blood pressure
- Feeling lightheaded or dizzy
- Shortness of breath
- Weakening or noticeable increase of pulse

Food allergies and bee stings are the most likely cause of severe reactions that can be fatal. People who have been diagnosed with severe allergies often carry an EpiPen – or similar shot – that helps stop the reaction before it becomes fatal.

Allergy Development

Typically, to develop an allergy, the person must first come in contact with the foreign substance. Allergies are, essentially, a learned reaction that the immune system develops over a period of time. This reaction can start out small and become more extreme as time passes.

Allergies and allergy-related diseases are on the rise, especially in developed nations, according to the World Allergy Organization. The cause of this increase is currently being researched and should be taken seriously. The World Allergy Organization has also found that there is an increase in dangerous symptoms suffered by children. Because of this, most schools have bared children from bringing any foods to school that contain nuts. This is to protect the children who suffer from a potentially fatal allergy to nuts.

Allergies can also lead to another problem, the development of serious illnesses. Respiratory allergies, for example, are a common allergy that many people think little about and take a casual approach to them. Unfortunately, someone with respiratory allergies can develop asthma due to the constant irritation that the respiratory system suffers. Eczema is another illness that can be caused by allergies.

Even if you're allergies are a mere annoyance, they will usually get worse with time. That is why you should try to identify the causes of any reactions you have. Doing so will help you avoid prolonged exposure to the substance that is causing your body to react in such a negative way.

Chapter 3 – Best Essential Oils for Treating Allergies

While there are an abundance of essentials oils that can be used to relieve allergies, the following are essential oils that experts generally classify as the most effective for allergies.

Clary Sage

Clary sage (Salvia sclaria) is a member of the mint family.

It provides many benefits, including de-stressing and relaxation properties. This can come in handy when you're allergies cause you to wheeze and sneeze like crazy. Clary sage is a mellow, warm and relaxing herb that naturally contains phytoestrogens. It is frequently used to support positive thoughts and attitudes. Clary sage is also a common herb used to treat symptoms associated with menstrual cycles and menopause, such as cramps and mood changes. Clary sage has balancing and calming properties that can quiet the mind. This essential oil is also a natural astringent, antidepressant, digestive, aphrodisiac, sedative, stomachic and hypotensive, among others. Furthermore, clary sage is known as a good eye cleanser, can help protect eyesight loss due to natural aging and even improve vision.

Clove Oil

Clove essential oil has a sweet yet spicy aroma and is used to treat various ailments, including supporting healthy digestive and immune systems. The revitalizing and stimulating effect of clove oil means it can help energize the spirit, body and mind. Historically, clove oil has been used to relieve dental issues (because it contains eugenol, which is a numbing agent), sinus problems and head conditions. Clove oil has antioxidant properties and is rich in vitamin A, vitamin C, potassium, hydrochloric acid, calcium and iron.

Cypress Oil

Cypress essential oil have a fresh, evergreen-like aroma, and is considered to be a stabilizing grounding and soothing oil that can help keep those bad feelings at bay during the winter months. It also naturally soothes the sinuses and nose. The compounds found in cypress oil have medicinal-like properties that can treat various discomforts and ailments, including allergies. Cypress is a disinfectant that actually prevents bacterial infections from forming in the sinus membranes. It also has anti-inflammatory and antispasmodic, and can suppress coughing and other symptoms associated with asthmatics.

Frankincense Essential Oil

For thousands of years, this essential oil has been used to treat a number of aliments. In fact, it is one that you should keep on hand at all times. Not only is it good for treating allergies, but it is also a natural antiseptic and disinfectant.

Lemongrass Essential Oil

While lemongrass essential oil is typically used as a natural pain reliever, it contains antibacterial properties, which is important for people who suffer from sinus problems and allergies. Furthermore, lemongrass has a pleasant citrusy aroma that fills the air.

Eucalyptus Essential Oil

Known for its respiratory system benefits, eucalyptus essential oil is a potent decongestant, antiseptic and anti-inflammatory. All traits that are ideal for treating allergies.

Ginger Essential Oil

Nausea is a common symptoms of an intense sinus attack, and ginger essential oil helps to get rid of your uneasy stomach. Ginger also contains anti-inflammatory and antibacterial compounds, and have a calming effect on the stomach and nervous system.

Lemon Essential Oil

Lemon essential oil isn't just useful because of its pleasant citrusy scent; it also has natural medicinal value. This essential oil has anti-infection properties, which make it ideal for those suffering from sinus problems since infection is common. Lemon essential oil has acts as an antifungal, antiseptic, detoxifier and disinfectant.

Peppermint Essential Oil

Known for its natural anti-inflammatory and pain reliving properties, peppermint can help relieve nasal and respiratory congestion.

Roman Chamomile Essential Oil

Known for its natural calming effect, Roman chamomile essential oil has been used for years to treat a wide array of health problems, including allergies. It has anti-inflammatory, anti-parasitic and anti-infectious properties. Furthermore, Roman chamomile can help relax emotions and nervous systems.

Rosemary Essential Oil

Rosemary has a wide array of health benefits, including the ability to boost mental activity, stimulate hair growth, reduce pain and help relieve respiratory problems. It has anti-inflammatory, stress relieving and antibacterial properties. It is also known as a natural disinfectant that can help remove bacteria from the throat and nose.

Tea Tree Essential Oil

No matter what, tea tree oil should be in your essential oil arsenal bag. It can help relieve intense sneezing, sniffles and various other symptoms associated with allergies. Tea tree has antiseptic, antibacterial, cicatrisant, antimicrobial, balsamic, expectorant, fungicide and insecticide properties.

Lavender Essential Oil

Like tea tree, lavender essential oil should be kept on hand at all times. This vestal oil has a cornucopia of benefits for your health. In fact, lavender is one of the most versatile of all the other essential oils. Lavender not only clams the nerves, but it also acts as a natural stamina and energy booster.

Chapter 4 – Control Allergies Symptoms with Essential Oils

Eczema

Although not contagious, eczema is an unpleasant skin condition, which is also known as dermatitis. It is inflammatory and chronic, and can affect women, men and children alike. This condition prevents the skin from producing the proper amount of oils and fats, which will reduce the skin's ability to retain water. This causes gaps to form, which results in moisture loss from deep in the skin's layers that, in turn, allows irritants to penetrate the skin.

Eczema typically causes itchy rashes or thick, scaly patches to form on the skin. They can occur on various parts of the body, including the cheeks, forehead, arms, elbows, legs and knees.

Common symptoms of eczema include redness, itchiness, dryness, crusting, swelling, cracking, flaking, oozing, bleeding and blisters of the skin.

Allergies, genetic or environmental factors triggers this condition, and must people suffering from it will generally use over the counter creams to help achieve relief. Unfortunately, these creams are not only filled with unnecessary chemicals, they do little to treat the condition, which will only become more severe. You can, however, find relief while treating the condition with the following homemade eczema cream recipe that doesn't contain harsh and potentially harmful ingredients.

Essential Oils for Eczema

Managing and treating eczema can be done with essential oils, which can be applied topically or as a skin cooling compress, in baths, as massage oil and a skin-cooling spray.

The following essential oils have proven to be effective on eczema.

Lavender Essential Oil

Lavender is an all-purpose oil that has a number of health benefits. It has natural anti-inflammatory, antibacterial, antifungal, antiseptic and moisturizing properties. Because of these properties, lavender essential oil can prevent skin scarring and speed up the healing process. Apply diluted lavender essential oil topically up to three times a day until the skin heals.

Tea Tree Essential Oil

This versatile oil has anti-inflammatory, antiviral, antibacterial and antiseptic properties, which makes it great for healing eczema, as well as other skin disorders.

German or Roman Chamomile Essential Oil

Known for their anti-inflammatory properties, German and Roman chamomile essential oil is great for managing and treating eczema. The natural properties found in these two chamomile essential oils are also good for soothing itchy and dry skin patches and reducing skin inflammation caused by eczema.

Thyme Essential Oil

Thyme has an energizing fragrance that contains a wide array of properties useful for treating eczema, including antibacterial, antioxidant, antifungal and antiviral.

Hay Fever

A collection of symptoms, hay fever is the allergic reaction to pollen. Those suffering from hay fever usually will also suffer from other allergic conditions, such as allergic asthma and atopic dermatitis. Furthermore, the chance for people suffering from hay fever to develop asthmatic attacks increases.

The symptoms must commonly associated with hay fever are itchy throat, runny nose, itchy eyes, perennial sneezing, itchy nose, red eyes and possible conjunctivitis. Itching will generally occur first, followed by sneezing, congestion and runny nose. However, the cause and effects of hay fever are rarely the same in two people. Because of this, the effective remedies to treat hay fever will vary from one person to the next.

Hay fever occurs most often in the flowering season, and can occur, in one form or another, in the spring, summer and autumn.

Lavender essential oil, German chamomile essential oil, chamomile essential oil, Melissa essential oil, lemon essential oil, peppermint essential oil, clove essential oil and yarrow essential oil are the most common essential oils used to control and treat hay fever.

Massaging a mixture of five drops lavender essential oil and two teaspoons of carrier oil into the sinus area (located below your eyes) will effectively alleviate a hay fever attack. Another option is to blend two drops eucalyptus, two drop German chamomile, two drops lavender, two drops lavender, two drops lemon and two drops balm essential oil together. Dampen a clean handkerchief into the blend. Cover your nose and mouth with the handkerchief and inhale.

Known for building your immune resistance to hay fever, yarrow essential oil can help prevent attacks. Simply consume four or more drops of yarrow essential oil in the desired formula. For best results, start about two weeks before hay fever season begins.

Itchy Eyes

Considered an acute eye problem for many, itchy eyes produce a hive-like reaction when the eyes are exposed to any foreign particles. While foreign particles are the leading cause of itchy eyes, winds – be it hot or cold winds – are another cause of this unpleasant condition.

The most common symptoms of itchy eyes include red, inflamed or swollen eyes. Itchy eyes may or may not be accompanied by scaly, dry dermatitis.

Lavender, frankincense, peppermint, melaleuca, eucalyptus and helichrysum are a few of the essential oils that can help alleviate itchy eyes.

Mold Allergies

Mold allergies occur when you inhale mold spores, which are microscopic particles that can be found both inside and outside the home. Allergic reaction can also occur if the mold spores comes in contact with your eyes.

Mold spores can be found anywhere in the home, but generally occur in damp areas, such as bathrooms, basements and closets. Essentially, mold can form anywhere there is moisture. Outdoors, mold can be found in garbage cans, wood piles, underneath floor mats, freshly mowed grass, air conditioning systems, poorly drained areas and camping equipment, among other places.

Mold spores can enter your home from the outside via windows, doors and air leaks. However, diagnosing mold allergies may be tricky because the symptoms are similar to various other common allergies. The symptoms of mold allergies include sneezing, runny nose, postnasal drip and coughing.

Peppermint, lavender, frankincense, Roman chamomile, lemongrass, tea tree, rosewood, geranium rose and lemon essential oil are all recommended to treat symptoms associated with mold allergies.

Atopic Dermatitis
When skin is sensitive to allergens, the pruritic condition known as atopic dermatitis will occur. This recurring and chronic condition makes the

skin red, itchy and flaky. These patches will often become flaky and dry, and may even ooze.

Atopic dermatitis results from parasitic invasion, genetics, emotional stress and allergy development, such as hay fever, asthma and rhinitis. The symptoms associated with this condition will disappear just to recur later on. While the disease itself currently has no known treatment, you can manage the symptoms to help reduce its severity. Those suffering from atopic dermatitis are typically prescribed topical and oral corticosteroids, antihistamines and antibiotics. However, many people choose to use essential oils to control atopic dermatitis symptoms because of the potential toxicity the prescribed medication can have.

Essential Oils for Atopic Dermatitis

The ideal essential oils for use on atopic dermatitis are those that have soothing and anti-inflammatory properties. A carrier oil –

such as jojoba oil or extra-virgin olive oil – should be used to help increase the essential oil's soothing capability.

German Chamomile Essential Oil
This is one of the best essential oils for use on atopic dermatitis because of its soothing, anti-inflammatory and anti-allergic properties. To use, simply dilute three or four drops of the essential oil with your desired carrier oil. Soak a clean gauze in the mixture. Apply the gauze directly to the affected areas of skin.

Lavender Essential Oil
Known for its stress reducing, balancing, cell regenerative, anti-infectious, skin tonic and soothing properties, lavender essential oil is a wonderful way to help combat symptoms associated with atopic dermatitis. A few drops of lavender essential oil added to bath water will help soothe the affected areas.

Frankincense Essential Oil

This beneficial essential oil has shown to have anti-inflammatory, wound healing and anti-infectious properties, which makes it great for relieving symptoms associated with atopic dermatitis.

Helichrysum Essential Oil
This beneficial essential oil anti-inflammatory, scar reduction and cell regenerative properties, which come in handy when dealing with atopic dermatitis.

Cedarwood Essential Oil
This essential oil has shown to be useful when trying to manage atopic dermatitis symptoms. It can help improve the autonomic balance of the body and acts as a gentle circulatory stimulant.

Rosemary Essential Oil
Rosemary is well known for its cell regenerative, scar reduction and anti-infectious properties, which are all important when trying

to manage the symptoms associated with atopic dermatitis.

Bags and Dark Circles under Eyes

While bags and dark circles are not a serious concern, they can make you appear older than you are. And they are, unfortunately, a common side effect of allergies. When the skin underneath the eyes becomes thinner and transparent, bags and dark circles will appear. This is because the blood-filled veins located under the eye makes the skin look darker.

Hay fever and asthma are two common allergies that can lead to bags and/or dark circles to appear under the eyes. Thankfully, there are a few essential oils that will help you effectively treat bags and dark circles. These essential oils include:

- Lemon essential oil
- Lavender essential oil
- Chamomile essential oil
- Rose essential oil

- Eucalyptus essential oil
- Almond essential oil
- Sandalwood essential oil

Rose and sandalwood essential oil helps to rejuvenate and hydrate the skin, while chamomile improves the overall quality of sleep, thus reducing the appearance of bags and dark circles. Almond essential oil is rich in vitamin K, which is vital for getting rid of skin discoloration and dark circles.

Eucalyptus Essential Oil – Dilute 3 to 4 drops with a carrier oil and massage gently into the affected area. Leave on for 15-minutes before washing the essential oil off.

Almond Essential Oil – Before bed, massage diluted almond essential oil into the affected areas. In the morning, wash your face as you normally would. Repeat for several days until the bags and dark circles disappear.

Rose and Sandalwood Essential Oil – Steam water in a medium-sized bowl and add a few drops of the oils individually. Hold your head over the steaming water and cover your head with a towel. This will keep the steam directed at your face.

Cat and Dog Allergies

People of all ages, gender and walks of life can develop cat and/or dog allergies. Those suffering from cat and dog allergies typically also have mild to moderate allergies to pollen. They also tend to be allergic to the urine, dander or saliva of the animal.

The allergens that cats produce that cause allergies are found in their skin, fur and/or saliva. Symptoms of cat allergies include wheezing, sneezing, itchy red eyes, hives and nasal congestion. Dogs produce allergens located in their urine, salvia, dander and hair. Symptoms of dog allergies include water eyes, sneezing, itchy eyes, coughing, nasal congestion, hives and running nose.

Treatment for cat and dog allergies vary on the symptoms that are present. Eye problems, for example, are generally treated with eye drops containing antihistamine, while antihistamines or steroid nasal sprays are used to treat nasal problems. Some doctors even recommend getting an allergy shot to help build up tolerance. You can also use essential oils to help alleviate the symptoms associated with cat and dog allergies.

Lavender Essential Oil - Lavender essential oil has many different therapeutic benefits and is often known as a natural antihistamine. And since it is safe to ingest, you can add a few drops of lavender essential oil into a gelatin capsule. Lavender essential oil can also be used topically, even on sensitive skin. In addition, you can add a few drops of lavender essential oil to a bowl of hot water, and then –

while covering your head with a towel – place your head down toward the bowl to inhale the steam.

Peppermint Essential Oil - The anti-inflammatory property of peppermint essential oil makes it ideal for naturally reducing inflammation that occurs from cat and dog allergies. You can use peppermint essential oil as a steam inhalation or in a diffuser. You can also apply the diluted oil to the area underneath your nose.

Lemon Essential Oil – When diffused at night, lemon essential oil is very helpful in reduce the symptoms associated with pet allergies. Alternatively, add a few drops of the undiluted oil directly to your pillow.

Food Allergies

Food allergies are caused by a wide array of food. In fact, there are almost two hundred different types of food allergies. The most common foods that can trigger allergies include:

- Tree nuts
- Shellfish
- Fish
- Eggs
- Wheat
- Soy
- Milk
- Peanuts

Allergies that are caused by vegetables or fruits are generally not as severe. With that said, it is not uncommon for someone to have an allergy to seeds, such as sesame seeds.

Symptoms of food allergies typically appear within a few minutes to 2 hours after the food has been consumed. These symptoms include hives, wheezing or coughing, rash or flushed skin, swelling of the throat and/or vocal cords, lightheadedness and/or dizziness, itchy or tingling sensation in the mouth, swelling of the tongue, lip or face, difficulty breathing, abdominal cramps, diarrhea and/or vomiting and loss of consciousness.

Essential oil experts generally recommend eucalyptus, rose, peppermint, lavender, chamomile, jasmine, fennel, Melissa and dill essential oil for managing symptoms associated with food allergies.

Diluted almond essential oil and sandalwood oil can be massaged into the back and abdomen area to help alleviate food allergies. It is best if this blend is warmed first and used when on an empty stomach. Another option is to apply one to two drops of peppermint essential oil, lavender essential oil or lemon essential oil directly to your tongue.

Sometimes, improperly digested protein can lead to food allergies flaring up. If this occurs, you can find relief with black pepper essential oil and juniper berry essential oil. When mixed together and massaged into your stomach, these two essential oils will help to increase stomach acid, thus reducing symptoms associated with food allergies.

Psoriasis

A non-contagious skin condition, psoriasis occurs because of an overactive immune system. It changes the life cycle of the skin cells, causing these cells to build up on the surface of the skin rapidly. Because of this, red, itchy and dry patches form on the skin.

Plaque psoriasis, scalp psoriasis, pustular psoriasis, nail psoriasis, inverse psoriasis, erthrodermic psoriasis, psoriatic arthritis and guttate psoriasis are the various types of this skin condition out there.

Factors such as immune system defects, environmental factors and genetic issues can all trigger psoriasis development. Psoriasis mainly affects areas where friction, trauma and rubbing occurs, such as the scalp, elbows and knees. Common symptoms associated with psoriasis are swollen and stiff joints, small spots on the skin that are red, scaling patches covered in silvery scales, cracked and bleeding skin. Nails may also be affected, becoming ridged or thickened and accompanied by a burning or itching sensation.

There are several essential oils that can help treat and manage psoriasis. These oils include, thyme, lavender, Melrose, tea tree, geranium and sandalwood.

Thyme essential oil contains antiseptic properties that can help naturally treat various skin conditions, such as psoriasis. Dilute thyme with a carrier oil and apply topically to the affected area. Keep in mind, however, that thyme essential oil should not be used if pregnant or have high blood pressure.

The anti-inflammatory, antifungal, antiseptic and analgesic properties of lavender essential oil make it an effective treatment against the itchiness, secondary infections and anxiety that occur with psoriasis. Lavender essential oil can be applied topically to the psoriasis patches, inhaled or diffuse.

Melrose essential oil is a topical antiseptic that is commonly used to clean rashes and bruises. The anti-inflammatory properties found in Melrose can regenerate damaged skin tissue and reduce inflammation. Dilute Melrose essential oil with carrier oil and apply topically to the affected areas.

Tea tree essential oil is the go-to oil for a lot of skin conditions, including psoriasis. This is because it is rich in cell regenerative and anti-inflammatory properties. Use the oil undiluted in a diffuser or diluted and applied topically.

Sandalwood essential oil has numerous beneficial properties that can help treat and manage psoriasis. It's ability to relieve inflammation makes it useful for treating psoriasis flare-ups. Sandalwood can be diffused or applied in a diluted form to the affected skin.

Sinus Headache

When the sinuses become inflamed, a painful sinus headache will occur. But why does inflammation occur in the sinus cavities? Well, the actual condition is called sinusitis, which is just a fancy name for a congested and inflamed sinus cavity. When the sinuses are inflamed, the mucus draining areas become blocked, which prevents the mucus from draining out. This will create the perfect environment for bacteria, viruses and fungus that can lead to infections. Hay fever, colds and environmental factors are common culprits of sinusitis. The headaches associated with this condition occur because of an increase in the inflammatory fluid and a decrease in the mucus drainage.

The major symptoms of sinus headache are, of course, pain and pressure. Pain can become even more severe when the head is moved or bent forward suddenly or during temperature changes. Other symptoms include, painful pressure and tenderness of the face. With that said, symptoms associated with sinus headaches can be related to a sinus inflammation. And sinus inflammation symptoms include fever, fatigue, postnasal drip with a sore throat and a runny nose with green discharge.

Eucalyptus essential oil contains oxide 1, 8-cineole, which is an expectorant and anti-inflammatory. Because of this, eucalyptus is recommended at treating sinus headaches.

Roman chamomile is widely known for its sedative and anti-inflammatory properties. This oil can be used at night or in the evening to ease symptoms associated with sinus headaches.

Lavender essential oil, as I am sure you are aware of by now, has sedative and anti-inflammatory properties, which make it wonderful for relieving sinus headaches. For best results, use lavender in the evening or at night.

Spearmint essential oil is one of the best mint oils for treating sinus headaches. This is because of the abundance of menthol it contains without the typical strong aroma associated with mints. Peppermint essential oil is also effective at alleviating tension and pain associated with sinus headaches.

Hives (Urticaria)

Commonly known as hives, urticaria is an allergic skin condition that causes patches of red, itchy blisters to appear on the skin. These patches occur when blood plasma leaks into the skin. And this leakage is due to excessive histamine. Hives can be either chronic or acute.

Hives are the body's response to irritants or allergens, such as food (like diary, chocolate, soya and nuts), paint fumes, dust, insect bites, soap and pollen. Triggers like pet dander, emotional stress, temperature ranges, immune balance skin stimulus and viral or bacterial infections can also result in hives.

When looking for essential oils for hives you must choose one that has antihistamine, anti-inflammatory, soothing, antiseptic, antibacterial and antimicrobial properties. Lavender, chamomile, peppermint and helichrysum are a few of the essential oils that fit the bill when it comes to treating hives.

Chapter 5 – Essential Oil Recipes that Treat Allergies

Eczema Cream Recipe

Ingredients:

- ¼ cup shea butter
- ¼ cup coconut oil, melted or soft
- ½ teaspoon vitamin E oil
- 15 drops lavender essential oil
- 25 drops Melrose essential oil

Directions:

Step 1: Mix the shea butter, coconut oil and vitamin E oil together in a small bowl. Stir thoroughly until well combined.

Step 2: Add the essential oils to the mixture one drop at a time. Stir until the oils are well incorporated.

Step 3: Scoop the cream out of the bowl and into a container. Store at room temperature. Keep in mind, however, that the cream may become a bit melty if kept in an area with temperatures higher than 75-degrees. In this case, you can place the cream in the fridge.

Step 4: When ready to use, rub the cream into the skin suffering from eczema.

Simple Eczema-Healing Skin Cream

Ingredients:

- ½ cup coconut oil
- 25 drops lavender essential oil
- 25 drops Melrose essential oil

Directions:

Step 1: Fill a small pot with water and bring to a simmer over medium-low heat.

Step 2: Add the coconut oil to a pint-sized Mason jar. Set the oil-filled Mason jar inside the water-filled pot. Heat until the oil has liquefied.

Step 3: Remove the Mason jar from heat and let cool for a couple of minutes while stirring.

Step 4: Add the essential oils to the melted coconut oil when it has cooled to touch.

Step 5: Secure the lid onto the Mason jar and let cool. As it comes to room temperature, the cream will begin to solidify.

Lotion for Eczema

Ingredients:

- ½ cup shea butter
- 30 drops cedarwood essential oil
- 20 drops geranium essential oil
- 20 drops lavender essential oil

Directions:

Step 1: Place the shea butter in a mixing bowl. Use a hand whisk to whip the shea butter into the light and fluffy consistency.

Step 2: Add the cedarwood, geranium and lavender essential oil to the shea butter.

Step 3: Whisk the shea butter and essential oils together with the hand whisk until well mixed.

Step 4: Transfer the lotion into the desired container.

Step 5: When ready to use, massage a bit of the lotion onto trouble spots.

Eczema Scar Healing Lotion
Ingredients:
- 1 ounce coconut oil
- 8 drops lemongrass essential oil
- 10 drops geranium essential oil
- 6 drops lavender essential oil
- 3 drops melrose essential oil
- 3 drops frankincense essential oil

Directions:
Step 1: Bring a pot of water to a simmer on the stove. Set a heatproof glass bowl on top of the pot.
Step 2: Place the coconut oil into the glass bowl. Let the coconut oil melt slowly over the simmering water.
Step 3: Remove the glass bowl from heat and let cool a bit. The coconut oil should be warm to the touch but not hot.

Step 4: Stir in the lemongrass, geranium, lavender, melrose and frankincense essential oil.

Step 5: Spoon the healing scar lotion into an airtight glass jar. Place the jar in the fridge to allow the lotion to firm. Apply to scars twice a day to help speed healing and reduce their appearance

Rash Eczema and Psoriasis Lotion

Ingredients:

- 2 ounces shea butter
- 2 tablespoons sweet almond oil
- 1 tablespoon beeswax
- 10 drops German chamomile essential oil
- 10 drops lavender essential oil
- 10 drops vitamin E oil

Directions

Step 1: Place the shea butter, sweet almond oil and beeswax in a double boiler. Melt the three ingredients together while stirring continuously throughout the process.

Step 2: Remove the melted mixture from heat and let to the touch.

Step 3: Stir in the German chamomile essential oil, lavender essential oil and vitamin E oil.

Step 4: Transfer the lotion to an airtight glass jar. Let the lotion cool completely before use.

Maximum Strength Lotion for Psoriasis and Eczema

Ingredients:

- ½ tablespoons emulsifying wax
- ½ teaspoon stearic acid
- 1/3 cup rosehip oil
- ½ cup distilled water
- 1 teaspoon vitamin E oil
- 10 drops grapefruit seed extract
- 1 tablespoon vegetable glycerin
- 4 drops frankincense essential oil
- 4 drops sandalwood essential oil
- 4 drops lavender essential oil
- 4 drops helichrysum essential oil
- 2 drops rose essential oil

- 2 drops chamomile essential oil

Directions:

Step 1: In a double boiler, melt the rosehip oil, emulsifying wax, vegetable glycerin and stearic acid. Make sure the ingredients are completely melted and the mixture is smooth.

Step 2: Remove the mixture from heat and stir in the vitamin E oil.

Step 3: Gently warm the distilled water in a small pot on the stove.

Step 4: Pour the warmed distilled water into the mixture from Step 1 and whisk thoroughly. Continue to whisk until the lotion mixture has a uniform color.

Step 5: Whisk in the grapefruit seed extract and the frankincense essential oil, sandalwood essential oil, lavender essential oil, helichrysum essential oil, rose essential oil and chamomile essential oil until thoroughly combined.

Step 6: Store the lotion into an airtight dark glass jar. Allow the lotion to cool completely before securing the lid on the jar.

All-Purpose Lavender Allergy Relief

Directions:

- *Topically*: Add 1 drop to your cheeks, forehead and sinuses as needed. Also, apply several drops to the soles of your feet before bed.

- *Diffuse*: Diffuse Lavender Essential Oil in a cold diffuser for 15 minutes every 2 hours. You can also diffuse beside your bed at night.

- *Inhalation*: Apply 1-2 drops of Lavender Essential Oil into the palms of your hands. After rubbing your hands together, cup them over your nose and deeply inhale 4-6 breaths. You can also place 2-3 drops on a cotton ball, secure it in a zip lock bag and take it with you. Inhale 4-6 breaths as needed.

Peppermint Nasal Decongestant

Directions:

- *Topically*: Apply 1 drop of Peppermint Essential Oil to the base of your neck 2 times daily. Also, dilute it in olive oil (or another carrier oil) and apply it around your nostrils. *WARNING: Do not apply this oil in full strength around nostrils as it will sting the sensitive tissues of the nostrils.

- *Diffuse*: Diffuse Peppermint Essential Oil by your bed and throughout the day. Follow directions of diffuser being used.
- *Inhalation*: Apply 1-2 drops in palm of your hand, rub your hands together and cup them over your nose. Inhale deeply 4-6 breaths. Also, you can place 2-3 drops on cotton ball, secure it in a zip lock bag and take it with you. Inhale 4-6 breaths as needed.

Lemon and Lavender Blend for Dark Circles and Bags

Ingredients:

- 1 drop lemon essential oil
- 1 drop lavender essential oil
- 1 teaspoon distilled water

Directions:

Step 1: Before bed, mix the lemon essential oil, lavender essential oil and distilled water together.

Step 2: Massage the blend into the skin underneath the eyes.

Step 3: In the morning, rinse your face with cool water.

Tummy Soothing Blend for Food Allergies

Ingredients:

- 5 drops chamomile essential oil
- 3 drops dill essential oil
- 2 drops ginger essential oil
- 2 drops peppermint essential oil
- 1 ounce carrier oil

Directions:

Step 1: Mix the essential oils and carrier oils together in small bowl.

Step 2: Massage the blend gently into the abdomen area.

Tip: Reduce the essential oil drops by half if using on a child.

Blend for Alleviating Food Allergies via Capsule

Ingredients:

- 2 drops lemon essential oil
- 2 drops peppermint essential oil
- 2 drops lavender essential oil
- 1 vegetable-base capsule

Directions:

Step 1: Mix the lemon, peppermint and lavender essential oils together in small bowl.

Step 2: Carefully open the capsule. Add the essential oils into the capsule and secure closed.

Step 3: Swallow the capsule with a glass of water. Repeat as needed at three hour intervals.

Combat Itchy Eye Blend #1

Ingredients:

- 3 drops lavender essential oil
- 2 drops melaleuca essential oil
- 5 drops coconut oil

Directions:

Step 1: Mix the three oils together in a small bowl.

Step 2: Gently massage the blend around your eye socket.

Step 3: Leave the blend on for several minutes before rinsing it off your skin.

Tip: Take care not to get the blend into your eyes as this will only lead to more problems.

Combat Itchy Eye Blend #2

Ingredients:

- 1 part eucalyptus essential oil
- 1 part frankincense essential oil
- 1 part peppermint essential oil

Directions:

Step 1: Mix the three oils together in a small bowl.

Step 2: Gently massage the blend around your eye socket.

Step 3: Leave the blend on for several minutes before rinsing it off your skin.

Tip: Take care not to get the blend into your eyes as this will only lead to more problems.

Mold Allergy Diffusing Blend #1

Ingredients:

- 3 drops Roman chamomile essential oil
- 3 drops rosewood essential oil
- 3 drops geranium rose essential oil
- 10 drops lavender essential oil
- 8 ounces carrier oil

Directions:

Step 1: Mix all the oils together into a bowl.

Step 2: Transfer the blend to a diffuser. Diffuse the blend to relieve allergies. This blend has antihistamine properties that are successful for controlling mold allergies.

Mold Allergy Diffusing Blend #2

Ingredients:

- 3 drops thyme essential oil

- 3 drops ajowan essential oil
- 2 drops tea tree essential oil
- 2 drops oregano essential oil

Directions:

Step 1: Mix the thyme, ajowan, tea tree and oregano essential oil together in a bowl.

Step 2: Pour the mixture into a diffuser. Alternatively, use the blend as a steam inhalation.

Psoriasis-Relieving Blend for Bath

Ingredients:

- 1 part lavender essential oil
- 1 part bergamot essential oil
- 1 part German chamomile essential oil
- 1 part carrier oil

Directions:

Step 1: In a small bowl, mix all the oils together.

Step 2: Run a warm bath. Turn the water off and dump the oil blend directly into the bathwater. Use your hand to mix the oil blend and water together.

Step 3: Carefully submerge yourself into the warm water and soak for several minutes.

Step 5: Repeat the process two times a day to moisturize and soothe skin, while preventing infections.

Topical Psoriasis Blend

Ingredients:

- 1 part lavender essential oil
- 1 part ylang ylang essential oil
- 1 part geranium essential oil
- 1 part bergamot essential oil
- 1 part frankincense essential oil
- 1 part clary sage essential oil
- 2 parts carrier oil, such as sweet almond or avocado

Directions:

Step 1: Mix all the oils together in a small bowl.

Step 2: Gently massage the blend into the affected skin twice a day. For best results, apply with clean hands to clean skin.

Banish Sinus Headache Blend
Ingredients:
- 1 part peppermint essential oil
- 1 part spearmint essential oil
- 1 part chamomile essential oil
- 1 part eucalyptus essential oil
- 2 parts carrier oil

Directions:
Step 1: Combine the oils together in a bowl.
Step 2: Gently massage the oil blend into the neck, forehead and back to relieve sinus headache.

Steam Inhalation Blend for Sinus Headache
Ingredients:
- 1 part rosemary essential oil
- 1 part frankincense essential oil
- 1 part eucalyptus essential oil

Directions:

Step 1: Mix the three essential oils together.

Step 2: Prepare a steam inhalation with the oils. Relax and breathe in deeply during the steam inhalation process.

Step 3: Repeat the process twice a day to relieve sinus headache and pressure.

Hive-Relieving Bath Soak

Ingredients:

- 4 drops lavender essential oil
- 4 drops lemongrass essential oil
- 4 drops geranium essential oil

Directions:

Step 1: Fill a bathtub with warm water.

Step 2: Add the essential oils one drop at a time to the bathwater.

Step 3: Submerge yourself into the warm water and soak for at least 15 minutes. The essential oil blend will help relieve the symptoms associated with hives.

Anti-Itch Hive Treatment

Ingredients:

- 1 part chamomile essential oil
- 1 peppermint essential oil

Directions:

Step 1: Mix the chamomile and peppermint essential oil together.

Step 2: Dampen a clean cloth in the blend. Press the cloth to the affected area.

Step 3: Keep the cloth on the skin for several minutes to alleviate itching caused by hives.

Massage Blend for Hives

Ingredients:

- 1 part helichrysum essential oil
- 1 part melaleuca essential oil
- 1 part frankincense essential oil

Directions:

Step 1: Mix the three essential oils together in a small bowl.

Step 2: Massage the blend into the affected areas three times a day to relieve symptoms associated with hives.

Chapter 6 – Tips and Tricks for Proper Essential Oil Use

Tip #1: When mixing essential oils with a carrier oil, you should pour half of the carrier oil into the desired container and then add all the essential oils. Finish it off by adding the remaining amount of carrier oil. This will ensure that you have room for the essential oils, which are the most important part of the recipe.

Tip #2: When you are pouring the oils – be it essential oils or carrier oil – into the desired storage container, leave a bit of space at the top of the container. This will let the oils breathe.

Tip #3: When mixing essential oils, do so gently. Rapid stirring or vigorous shaking can actually damage the organic, delicate compounds that make the essential oil beneficial. Furthermore, exposing essential oils to excessive light or heat can change their composition and make them spoil and oxidize quicker.

Tip #4: You should only use glass, ceramic or plastic tools when working with essential oils. Never use anything metal!

Tip #5: A little essential oil goes a long way. And you should remember this if you are using essential oils for skin care. What does this mean exactly? Well, it means that you don't need to use an abundance of the oils. For example, a few drops will usually be enough to treat your whole face.

Tip #6: Not every essential oil is safe for use on children or women who are either pregnant or nursing. That is why you should always consult with a medical professional before using any essential oil.

Tip #7: You should always perform an allergy test before using any essential oil on your body. This can be done by applying one or two drops of the essential oil (or essential oil blend) to the back of your hand. If, however, after several hours no adverse effects have occurred, you can use the essential oil as desired.

Tip #8: All citrus essential oils may cause photosensitivity when exposed to the sun. So, if you are using any essential oil or blend that contains citrus, you should apply it only at night or when you won't be in the sunlight that day. In fact, you shouldn't apply it within 12 hours of sun exposure.

Chapter 7 – Essential Oil Safety

While essential oils are generally thought of as a safer option to potentially harmful and toxic prescriptions, safety is still an issue. These powerful oils are actually concentrated, which can lead to serious damage to your health if not used properly and responsibly. To show you just how concentrated these oils are; it takes a whopping 256 pounds of peppermint leaves to get a mere 1 pound of its essential oil. Now that is some powerfully concentrated oil! Because of the high level of concentration, you really only need to use a small amount of the oil. Furthermore, almost all essential oils should be diluted if it will come in contact with the skin.

Photosensitivity

Some essential oils – such as orange, lemon, lime, grapefruit and bergamot – cause the skin to become more sensitive to sunlight (UV light). This condition is known as photosensitivity and can cause blistering and discoloration to the skin. It can also leave your skin more susceptible to burning from the sun. In order to avoid photosensitivity, never apply essential oils known to cause this problem within a 12 hour period when your skin will become exposed to sunlight.

Babies and Children

Most experts would suggest avoid using essential oils on babies and children unless you get the okay from a trusted doctor. If you do use essential oils are your little ones, always exercise extreme caution and dilute the oils more so than you would for an adult. The skin of babies and children are more sensitive than that of an adult, and essential oils that are safe can actually damage their skin. However, there are a few essential oils that experts agree are safe, if used properly, for use on babies and children. These oils include chamomile, lavender, frankincense, lemon and orange. With that said, you should never use peppermint, eucalyptus, wintergreen or rosemary essential oil on babies and children.

Pregnancy or Nursing

Essential oils should be avoided when pregnant or nursing. This is because essential oils have shown to have an effect on hormones, gut bacteria and various other important body aspects that may be harmful or dangerous to the baby in the womb. If, however, you decide to go ahead and use essential oils during this time, you must always proceed with extreme caution. And never use any essential oils without first getting the okay from your doctor.

With that said, there are several oils that experts agree are not safe for use at any time during pregnancy. Rosemary, sage, cinnamon, basil, angelica, black pepper, aniseed, clary sage, chamomile, camphor, clove, fennel, ginger, horseradish, mustard, jasmine, juniper, nutmeg, mugwart, peppermint, marjoram, myrrh, thyme and wintergreen are among the essential oils that pregnant women should avoid at all cost.

A good general rule of thumb is to talk to your doctor or midwife about essential oils before using if pregnant or nursing. They will be able to give you their expert opinion on whether or not an essential oil should be used.

Conclusion

Thank you again for reading this book!

I hope this book was able to help you learn more about essential oils and how they can help relief, treat and manage your allergies.

Keep in mind, however, that not every brand of essential oil is created equal and you should always aim to use high quality oils from a reputable merchant. Furthermore, you should only use therapeutic grade or organic 100-percent pure essential oils. These oils are created using non-chemical process – such as steam distillation – and are considered safe to use both internally and externally.

If you got this far you are one of the few people who take actions. Please leave us a review on Amazon.com